Copyright ©2020
RND
All rights reserved. No part of this publication may be reproduced, distributed, or transmitted in any form or by any means, including photocopying, recording, or other electronic or mechanical methods, without the prior written permission of the publisher, except in the case of brief quotations embodied in critical reviews and certain other noncommercial uses permitted by copyright law.

Contents

- INTRODUCTION 5
  - Symptoms 6
    - When To See A Doctor 7
  - Causes 7
  - Risk Factors 8
  - Complications 9
  - Diagnosis 10
  - Imaging tests 11
  - Laboratory tests 11
  - Treatment 12
  - Medications 12
  - Surgical and other procedures 14
  - Lifestyle And Home Remedies 15
  - Preparing for your appointment 17
  - What you can do 18
  - What to expect from your doctor 18
    - What joints are affected 19
  - Myths About Psoriatic Arthritis Treatment 19
  - Special Diet To Help You Manage Psoriatic Arthritis ... 27
  - Mediterranean Diet 28
  - Why might it be good for psoriatic arthritis 29
  - Paleolithic Diet 30

- Why might it be good for psoriatic arthritis 31
  - Vegetarian or Vegan Diet 32
  - Why might it be good for psoriatic arthritis 33
- Gluten-Free Diet 34
  - Why might it be good for psoriatic arthritis 35
- Pagano Diet 36
  - Why might it be good for psoriatic arthritis 36
  - Things to Keep in Mind for Any Psoriatic Arthritis Diet 38
- Psoriasis Arthritis Recipes 39
  - Trail Mix 39
  - Greens Smoothie 41
  - Yogurt Sundae 42
  - Almond Flour Cakes 43
  - Baked Rainbow Trout 45
  - Baked Chicken 46
  - Gluten-Free Bean Salad 48
  - Salad Dressing 49
  - Broccoli and Barley Soup 56
  - Chicken Soup with Rice and Broccoli 58
  - Romaine and Smoked Salmon Salad 61
  - Beet and Carrot Salad with Ginger 62
  - Beet and Carrot Soup 63
  - Omega-3 Omelet with Red Onions and Capers 64

Barley Soup with Carrots and Parsley 65

Conclusion 66

INTRODUCTION

Psoriatic arthritis is most commonly a seronegative oligoarthritis found in patients with psoriasis, with less common, but characteristic, differentiating features of distal joint involvement and arthritis mutilans. One in five patients with psoriasis has psoriatic arthritis. Psoriatic arthritis is a form of arthritis that affects some people who have psoriasis a condition that features red patches of skin topped with silvery scales. Most people develop psoriasis first and are later diagnosed with psoriatic arthritis, but the joint problems can sometimes begin before skin patches appear.

Joint pain, stiffness and swelling are the main signs and symptoms of psoriatic arthritis. They can affect any part of your body, including your fingertips and spine, and can range from relatively mild to severe. In both psoriasis and psoriatic arthritis, disease flares may alternate with periods of remission.

No cure for psoriatic arthritis exists, so the focus is on controlling symptoms and preventing damage to your joints. Without treatment, psoriatic arthritis may be disabling.

Symptoms

Both psoriatic arthritis and psoriasis are chronic diseases that get worse over time, but you may have periods when your symptoms improve or go into remission alternating with times when symptoms become worse.

Psoriatic arthritis can affect joints on just one side or on both sides of your body. The signs and symptoms of psoriatic arthritis often resemble those of rheumatoid arthritis. Both diseases cause joints to become painful, swollen and warm to the touch.

However, psoriatic arthritis is more likely to also cause:

Swollen fingers and toes. Psoriatic arthritis can cause a painful, sausage-like swelling of your fingers and toes. You may also develop swelling and deformities in your hands and feet before having significant joint symptoms.

Foot pain. Psoriatic arthritis can also cause pain at the points where tendons and ligaments attach to your bones especially at the back of your heel (Achilles tendinitis) or in the sole of your foot (plantar fasciitis).

Lower back pain. Some people develop a condition called spondylitis as a result of psoriatic arthritis. Spondylitis mainly causes inflammation of the joints between the vertebrae of your spine and in the joints between your spine and pelvis (sacroiliitis).

When To See A Doctor
If you have psoriasis, be sure to tell your doctor if you develop joint pain. Psoriatic arthritis can severely damage your joints if left untreated.

Causes
Psoriatic arthritis occurs when your body's immune system begins to attack healthy cells and tissue. The abnormal immune response causes inflammation in your joints as well as overproduction of skin cells.

It's not entirely clear why the immune system attacks healthy tissue, but it seems likely that both genetic and environmental factors play a role. Many people with psoriatic arthritis have a family history of either psoriasis or psoriatic arthritis. Researchers have discovered certain genetic markers that appear to be associated with psoriatic arthritis.

Physical trauma or something in the environment such as a viral or bacterial infection may trigger psoriatic arthritis in people with an inherited tendency.

Risk Factors
Thumbnails affected by psoriasis

Psoriasis on the nails Open pop-up dialog box

Several factors can increase your risk of psoriatic arthritis, including:

Psoriasis.

- Having psoriasis is the single greatest risk factor for developing psoriatic arthritis.
- People who have pitted, deformed nails are especially likely to develop psoriatic arthritis.
- Your family history. Many people with psoriatic arthritis have a parent or a sibling with the disease.
- Your age. Although anyone can develop psoriatic arthritis, it occurs most often in adults between the ages of 30 and 50.

Complications

A small percentage of people with psoriatic arthritis develop arthritis mutilans a severe, painful and disabling form of the disease. Over time, arthritis mutilans destroys the small bones in the hands, especially the fingers, leading to permanent deformity and disability.

People who have psoriatic arthritis sometimes also develop eye problems such as pinkeye (conjunctivitis) or uveitis, which can cause painful, reddened eyes and blurred vision. They are also at higher risk of cardiovascular disease.

Diagnosis
- During the exam, your doctor may:
- Closely examine your joints for signs of swelling or tenderness
- Check your fingernails for pitting, flaking and other abnormalities
- Press on the soles of your feet and around your heels to find tender areas
- No single test can confirm a diagnosis of psoriatic arthritis. But some types of tests can rule out other causes of joint pain, such as rheumatoid arthritis or gout.

Imaging tests

X-rays. Plain X-rays can help pinpoint changes in the joints that occur in psoriatic arthritis but not in other arthritic conditions.

Magnetic resonance imaging (MRI). MRI uses radio waves and a strong magnetic field to produce very detailed images of both hard and soft tissues in your body. This type of imaging test may be used to check for problems with the tendons and ligaments in your feet and lower back.

Laboratory tests

Rheumatoid factor (RF). RF is an antibody that's often present in the blood of people with rheumatoid arthritis, but it's not usually in the blood of people with psoriatic arthritis. For that reason, this test can help your doctor distinguish between the two conditions.

Joint fluid test. Using a needle, your doctor can remove a small sample of fluid from one of your affected joints often the knee. Uric acid crystals in your joint fluid may indicate that you have gout rather than psoriatic arthritis.

Treatment
No cure exists for psoriatic arthritis, so treatment focuses on controlling inflammation in your affected joints to prevent joint pain and disability.

Medications
Drugs used to treat psoriatic arthritis include:

NSAIDs. Nonsteroidal anti-inflammatory drugs (NSAIDs) can relieve pain and reduce inflammation. Over-the-counter NSAIDs include ibuprofen (Advil, Motrin IB, others) and naproxen sodium (Aleve). Stronger NSAIDs are available by prescription.

Side effects may include stomach irritation, heart problems, and liver and kidney damage.

Disease-modifying antirheumatic drugs (DMARDs). These drugs can slow the progression of psoriatic arthritis and save the joints and other tissues from permanent damage.

Common DMARDs include methotrexate (Trexall, Otrexup, others), leflunomide (Arava) and sulfasalazine (Azulfidine). Side effects vary but may include liver damage, bone marrow suppression and severe lung infections.

Immunosuppressants. These medications act to tame your immune system, which is out of control in psoriatic arthritis.

Examples include azathioprine (Imuran, Azasan) and cyclosporine (Gengraf, Neoral, Sandimmune). These medications can increase your susceptibility to infection.

Biologic agents. Also known as biologic response modifiers, this newer class of DMARDs includes abatacept (Orencia), adalimumab (Humira), certolizumab (Cimzia), etanercept (Enbrel), golimumab (Simponi), infliximab (Remicade), ixekizumab (Taltz), secukinumab (Cosentyx), tofacitinib (Xeljanz) and ustekinumab (Stelara).

These medications target specific parts of the immune system that trigger inflammation and lead to joint damage. These drugs can increase the risk of infections. Higher doses of tofacitinib can increase the risk of blood clots in the lungs. Biologic agents can be used alone or combined with DMARDs, such as methotrexate.

Newer oral medication. Apremilast (Otezla) decreases the activity of an enzyme in the body that controls the activity of inflammation within cells. Potential side effects include diarrhea, nausea and headaches.

Surgical and other procedures

Steroid injections. This type of medication reduces inflammation quickly and is sometimes injected into an affected joint.

Joint replacement surgery. Joints that have been severely damaged by psoriatic arthritis can be replaced with artificial prostheses made of metal and plastic.

Lifestyle And Home Remedies

Protect your joints. Changing the way you carry out everyday tasks can make a tremendous difference in how you feel.

For example, you can avoid straining your finger joints by using gadgets such as jar openers to twist the lids from jars, by lifting heavy pans or other objects with both hands, and by pushing doors open with your whole body instead of just your fingers.

Maintain a healthy weight. Maintaining a healthy weight places less strain on your joints, leading to reduced pain and increased energy and mobility. Losing weight if needed can also help your medications work better. Some psoriatic arthritis medications are less effective in people who have a body mass index of 25.0 to 29.9 (overweight).

The best way to increase nutrients while limiting calories is to eat more plant-based foods fruits, vegetables and whole grains.

Exercise regularly. Exercise can help keep your joints flexible and your muscles strong. Types of exercises that are less stressful on joints include biking, swimming and walking.

Stop smoking. Smoking is associated with a higher risk of developing psoriasis and with more-severe symptoms of psoriasis.

Limit alcohol use. Alcohol can increase your risk of psoriasis, decrease the effectiveness of your treatment and increase side effects from some medications, such as methotrexate.

Pace yourself. Battling pain and inflammation can leave you feeling exhausted. In addition, some arthritis medications can cause fatigue.

The key isn't to stop being active entirely, but to rest before you become too tired. Divide exercise or work activities into short segments. Find time to relax several times throughout the day.

Manage Stress To Improve Psoriatic Arthritis Symptoms

Psoriatic arthritis can be particularly discouraging because the emotional pain that psoriasis can cause is compounded by joint pain and, in some cases, disability.

The support of friends and family can make a tremendous difference when you're facing the physical and psychological challenges of psoriatic arthritis. For some people, support groups can offer the same benefits.

A counselor or therapist can help you devise coping strategies to reduce your stress levels. The chemicals your body releases when you're under stress can aggravate both psoriasis and psoriatic arthritis.

Preparing for your appointment

You're likely to first discuss your signs and symptoms with your family doctor. He or she may refer you to a doctor specializing in the treatment of arthritis and related disorders (rheumatologist).

What you can do

Before your appointment, you may want to write a list of answers to the following questions:

What types of symptoms are you having. When did they begin?

- Do you or any of your close family members have psoriasis?
- Has anyone in your immediate family ever had psoriatic arthritis?
- What medications and supplements do you take?
- You may want to bring a friend or a family member with you to your appointment. It's hard to remember everything about a complicated condition, and another person may remember information that you miss.

What to expect from your doctor

Your doctor might ask some of the following questions:

What joints are affected
- Are there any activities or positions that make your symptoms better or worse
- What treatments have you already tried. Have any of them helped.

Myths About Psoriatic Arthritis Treatment

Is there a cure for psoriatic arthritis. Can you stop treatment if you feel better. If you have psoriatic arthritis, it helps to study the condition so you can educate others about it. Joint pain, stiffness, swelling, fatigue for many people, aches and pains like these are just a part of getting older. But for about 30 percent of people with psoriasis, these symptoms may signal something more: psoriatic arthritis.

With psoriasis, joint pain may be a tip-off to psoriatic arthritis. And psoriatic arthritis treatment needs to be approached aggressively. The goal of psoriatic arthritis treatment is to relieve pain and inflammation and, if treatment begins early enough, prevent joint damage. People with psoriatic arthritis need to study their illness and be on top of it. That way, they can ask questions and be a real partner in the treatment process. Let's start by dispelling nine common misconceptions about psoriatic arthritis treatment.

Myth: It Doesn't Matter When You Start Treatment

When it comes to psoriatic arthritis, early diagnosis and treatment are critical. The earlier you catch it, the better chance you have to limit or even prevent joint damage from occurring, according to the NPF. Delay in diagnosis of as little as six months can lead to permanent joint damage.

What's more, early treatment of psoriatic arthritis can help preserve your ability to feel your best every day. The symptoms of joint pain and swelling are very limiting to people and can strongly influence quality of life. If you have psoriasis and believe you're experiencing arthritis-like symptoms, let your doctor know right away. You'll likely be referred to a rheumatologist, a doctor who specializes in arthritis.

Myth: Psoriatic Arthritis Is Curable

There's no cure for psoriatic arthritis. However, there are medications that can get it into remission. Treatment can help nearly 95 percent of people with different forms of arthritis start to feel better, and many people may also reach remission.

What does remission look like? Psoriatic arthritis remission can be defined as "the reversibility of functional impairment, minimal or no progression to joint destruction, and at least a theoretic potential to heal a damaged joint." For many people with psoriatic arthritis, reaching remission requires working closely with a doctor to find the appropriate treatment and then sticking to that treatment. Meanwhile, research for a psoriatic arthritis cure is under way.

Myth: A Dermatologist Can Treat Psoriatic Arthritis

Psoriasis and psoriatic arthritis are typically related, but that doesn't mean the approaches to treating and managing the conditions are identical. "Some people think, 'My psoriasis is doing well, so my arthritis isn't a big deal' or vice versa". The truth: "The two don't always correlate."

That's why it's important to also see a rheumatologist for psoriatic arthritis. In 85 percent of cases, skin problems occur before joint pain, so a dermatologist may be the first one to identify psoriatic arthritis. But because psoriatic arthritis treatment can be complex and often requires adjustments over time, a rheumatologist is best suited to develop your individual treatment plan. Sometimes treating one condition with certain medications may help improve the other.

Myth: NSAIDs Are Risk-Free

NSAIDs are commonly used to relieve joint pain, stiffness, and inflammation in people with psoriatic arthritis. Certain versions are available over the counter (like ibuprofen), while stronger forms require a prescription. For mild cases of psoriatic arthritis, NSAIDs can be helpful as they're for the management of pain. They don't change the course of the disease.

But just because NSAIDs are used for milder psoriatic arthritis symptoms, that doesn't mean they don't have risks or side effects. They do have risks. This can include stomach bleeding, hypertension, or kidney damage, especially if used at higher doses for long periods of time. Be sure to discuss these risks with your doctor.

Myth: Biologics and Newer Drugs Are Only for Severe Cases

Biologic drugs are disease-modifying, which means they stop or slow down disease by targeting specific parts of the immune system. Administered by injection or intravenous (IV) infusion, biologics also come with some risks.

In general, there's concern about any drug that modifies the immune system because of the possibility of infections or cancer development. While these concerns are valid, the benefits of biologic medications outweigh the risks, even for people whose cases are not severe. People who have mild pain or swelling in a single joint may do just fine with NSAIDs alone. For people who have more joint swelling and pain, the use of biologics is justified.

In addition, the newer oral treatment Otezla (apremilast) has been approved for active psoriatic arthritis as well as moderate to severe plaque psoriasis.

Myth: Long-Term Use of Corticosteroids Is Safe

At some point in the course of your disease, your doctor may prescribe a corticosteroid medication. According to the Psoriasis and Psoriatic Arthritis Alliance, low doses of corticosteroids may bring pain relief and ease stiffness in people with psoriatic arthritis, while higher doses can help with recovery from a severe flare-up.

But corticosteroid use is intended to be temporary. Because of the risk of serious side effects with long-term use such as muscle weakness, brittle bones, eye problems, and diabetes your doctor will only prescribe a corticosteroid when necessary and will likely taper you off it once the problem is under control.

Myth: You Can Stop Treatment When You Start Feeling Better

Most rheumatologists recommend that you stay on your medication even after you reach remission. We know that when people with psoriatic arthritis stop taking their medication, even if they feel good, their disease will come roaring back.

That only a small percentage of people with psoriatic arthritis who reach remission are able to stop taking their medication completely. Most people find that their disease flares up again. Indeed, a small study published found that about 77 percent of participants who stopped psoriatic arthritis treatment experienced a return of their symptoms within six months.

Myth: People With Psoriatic Arthritis Shouldn't Exercise

Wei and Matteson agree: If a person with psoriatic arthritis believes she shouldn't exercise because of joint pain, she may be falling for the biggest myth of all. Exercise should definitely be a part your overall treatment approach. Moderate physical activity may provide benefits for people with psoriatic arthritis by reducing joint pain and stiffness, improving flexibility, increasing range of motion, helping with weight loss, and more.

The most beneficial forms of physical activity for people with psoriatic arthritis tend to be walking, swimming, and biking. Exercises that strengthen muscle actually take stress off the joints. In addition to being good for your joints, fitness also plays an important role in your overall health.

Myth: Psoriatic Arthritis Eventually Requires Surgery

This myth is far from true. If psoriatic arthritis is diagnosed early and you are aggressive in treatment, you'll probably never need surgery. Only a small percentage of people with psoriatic arthritis will go on to require surgical intervention.

So who usually needs surgery. Some people have had the disease for many years before they start treatment, and severe joint destruction has already occurred. These people may undergo joint replacement surgery to relieve pain and restore function.

Special Diet To Help You Manage Psoriatic Arthritis

When it comes to living with psoriatic arthritis, eating a healthy, non-inflammatory diet can be an important part of managing your symptoms and feeling better. Maintaining a healthy weight is also important: Being overweight can make it harder to control symptoms, and obesity is linked to significantly higher disease severity. Rheumatic Diseases is just the latest to make this connection. The study of 917 people with psoriatic arthritis across eight European countries found that being overweight was associated with significantly higher psoriatic arthritis disease severity.

And while there's no scientific evidence that says eating a certain diet can have a significant and direct impact on psoriatic arthritis, some people have reported experiencing improvement in symptoms when they make some dietary changes. But regardless of how much your diet can impact your psoriatic arthritis, the fact is that eating a healthy diet can affect your overall health and reduce your risk of developing health problems that are related to psoriatic disease such as obesity, cardiovascular disease and diabetes.

Given this important possible connection, which diets are best for people who have psoriatic arthritis.

Mediterranean Diet
What it is:

While there isn't any one set definition of what constitutes a so-called Mediterranean diet, it's generally considered to be one that features fruits and vegetables, healthy fats (like olive oil), seafood, nuts, seeds, and legumes, and less red meat and carbohydrates than a typical American diet. (The name comes from the fact that countries in the Mediterranean region such as Italy, Spain, and Greece have followed this type of eating style for centuries.) There are also fewer sweets and desserts and butter in the Mediterranean diet.

Why might it be good for psoriatic arthritis

The Mediterranean diet is rich in omega-3 fatty acids, which are found in fish (especially cold-water fish that are high in fat such as salmon, mackerel, tuna, and sardines), nuts, and seeds (such as flaxseeds and chia seeds). Omega-3 fatty acids may help reduce inflammation and joint stiffness. And olive oil may also help arthritis: Olives and their derivatives (such as olive oil) have anti-inflammatory properties and may prevent cartilage damage due to osteoarthritis. And red meats and refined sugars, which are both considered inflammatory foods, are limited in this diet.

Generally speaking, the Mediterranean diet is a well-balanced diet. In contrast to the American diet, which is often loaded with fast foods and trans fats, the Mediterranean diet contains more fresh, whole foods. The more a food is processed, the less we know about what in that food might trigger inflammation and the less we are able to control an inflammatory condition [such as psoriatic arthritis].

Precautions for people with psoriatic arthritis:

While the Mediterranean diet is very healthy, there isn't a set amount of recommended fat or calories. The use of fat is not in a regulated amount, so it's important to watch how much you eat. The Mediterranean diet is not just a diet but also a lifestyle. Other aspects of the Mediterranean diet involves sharing meals with friends and family and being more physically active, which is a way of eating that is less likely to contribute to obesity.

Paleolithic Diet
What it is:

Also known as the paleo diet or the caveman diet, this dietary plan is modeled after what humans might have eaten some 2.5 million years ago, during the Paleolithic era. A typical paleo diet may include lean meats, fish, vegetables, fruits, nuts, and seeds foods that would've been obtained by hunting and gathering rather than farming. Foods that are not considered part of the paleo diet include grains (such as wheat, oats, and barley), legumes (beans, lentils, peas, and peanuts), dairy products, potatoes, and refined sugar, salt, and highly processed foods.

Why might it be good for psoriatic arthritis

It encourages food in its original form and not processed, and those who follow this diet tend to cook more. This diet, like the Mediterranean diet, is high in anti-inflammatory foods such as fish, nuts, seeds, fruits, and vegetables, and restricts foods thought to cause inflammation such as refined sugars, processed foods, and high-fat meat.

Precautions for people with psoriatic arthritis:

It lacks grains, dairy, and legumes so there's a lack of fiber, which keeps you regular and lowers your risk of cholesterol and diabetes. Constipation and bone health can be a concern. Lack of dairy may especially be problematic since psoriatic disease may increase your risk of osteoporosis. We need dairy to protect our bones. While some people with psoriatic arthritis report that eliminating dairy from their diet improves gastrointestinal symptoms (and there is a connection between inflammatory bowel disease and psoriatic arthritis, if you don't have trouble with dairy, eliminating it may not be beneficial and could risk bone health.

And while you may experience weight loss on the paleo diet which is a good thing for psoriatic arthritis management it may be due to the fact that whole categories of foods have been eliminated from the diet. There's a difference between removing a food that may cause symptoms and removing an entire food group.

Vegetarian or Vegan Diet
What it is:

Eating a vegetarian diet means eating a diet that focuses on plants (nuts, seeds, grains, fruits, vegetables) and occasionally includes dairy. A strictly vegetarian diet does not include meat or fish but some variations of a plant-based diet can include fish (pescatarian) or occasionally meat or poultry (semi-vegetarians). A vegan diet is one that excludes meat, poultry, fish, eggs, and dairy as well as anything that could be considered an animal product such as gelatin or honey.

Why might it be good for psoriatic arthritis

In a meta-analysis of 18 studies that evaluated effects of any type of vegetarian diet compared with omnivore diets on circulating levels of inflammatory biomarkers, following a vegetarian diet for at least two years was associated with lower levels of C-reactive protein, a key marker for inflammation in the body.

Precautions for people with psoriatic arthritis:

The concern with a vegetarian or vegan diet is whether or not someone is getting enough essential nutrients like protein, calcium, vitamin B12, and iron. When your body is lacking key nutrients, it requires a lot of work to make up for it and that can be a problem when you have a chronic condition such as psoriatic arthritis. You should maximize your diet to make sure your body always has good nutrition so that you can put all your energy to being healthy and managing your condition.

Gluten-Free Diet
What it is:

A gluten-free diet is one that cuts out foods that contain the protein gluten, which includes grains such as wheat, barley and rye. While a gluten-free diet is essential for people with conditions like celiac disease or a wheat allergy, there's been little solid medical evidence for removing gluten from the diet if you don't have a gluten sensitivity. Nevertheless, a gluten-free diet is one that's gained some popularity in recent years among people who do not have a diagnosed gluten intolerance. Some claimed benefits of a gluten-free diet are increased energy, weight loss, and improved overall health. There's a large discrepancy between what's reported and who actually cannot tolerate gluten. The reports of gluten intolerance are probably overinflated.

Why might it be good for psoriatic arthritis

Having an autoimmune condition like psoriatic arthritis increases the odds of having another autoimmune condition that some studies have linked psoriatic arthritis to an increased likelihood of developing celiac disease. There is a connection between psoriasis, psoriatic arthritis, and inflammatory bowel disease. Having psoriasis was associated with an increased risk of having Crohn's disease or ulcerative colitis.

While we don't yet have a clear understanding of this possible link, some people with psoriatic arthritis have reported having less joint pain after eliminating gluten from their diets.

Precautions for people with psoriatic arthritis:

If you have symptoms like diarrhea and constipation, you may want to talk to your doctor about trying out a gluten-free diet. But removing gluten from your diet requires working with a nutritionist or a doctor trained in nutrition to make sure you get adequate amounts of fiber and other nutrients and if it isn't something you need for a medical reason, it can be hard to stick to when you're on vacation, at work, or at school. You want a diet you can stick to for life.

Pagano Diet

This diet, created by a chiropractor named John O. A. Pagano, DC, is based upon the premise that all types of psoriasis are caused by a buildup of toxins in the intestines. The Pagano diet is mostly made up of fresh, organic fruits and vegetables and smaller amounts of wild meats and organic greens. It eliminates all red meat except lamb, all sweeteners, anything processed with preservatives or additives, and fried foods. It also eliminates white potatoes, chocolate, yeast, eggs, shellfish, citrus, and any nightshades (such as tomatoes, eggplant, and peppers).

Why might it be good for psoriatic arthritis

People with psoriatic disease reported that following certain diets, including the Pagano diet, was helpful for their symptoms. The researchers asked 1,200 NPF members about the influence of diet on their psoriasis symptoms and found that more than half of the study participants reported that they cut back on foods like alcohol, gluten, and nightshades and saw noticeable improvement of their symptoms. In addition to the Pagano diet, members reported other diets like the Mediterranean, gluten-free, and vegetarian diets to be helpful in managing their symptoms.

While there isn't solid evidence on whether any specific diet is most effective for psoriasis, there was one thing that has been shown to be beneficial is weight loss. While a certain diet might be worth trying with a doctor's supervision, losing weight has been shown to be effective for reducing stress on joints and decreasing inflammation.

Precautions for people with psoriatic arthritis:

As with any diet, it's essential that you work with a nutritionist to make sure that you aren't missing any key nutrients that you need for your body and mind to function properly. If you think you have an issue with a particular food, talk to your doctor or nutritionist about how to best eliminate it.

Things to Keep in Mind for Any Psoriatic Arthritis Diet

Regardless of which diet you choose, steer clear of inflammatory foods, says Bose. As a general rule, stay away from sugars, processed foods, and red meat and add beneficial foods such as fish, nuts, and seeds that are high in omega-3 fatty acids.

While weight loss is beneficial for psoriatic arthritis, losing too much might be a sign that you're missing something in your diet. Try to avoid switching eating patterns too much and too often. Drastic change to metabolism could be stressful to the body and could exacerbate inflammation. There is no one diet that's right for everyone with psoriatic arthritis. Every person is different. Someone may have a gluten intolerance while another might benefit from removing nightshades.

What you eat is only part of your psoriatic arthritis management. Making healthy lifestyle changes like exercising and talking to your doctor about other treatments is also part of disease management. Diet is a way to help symptoms and manage your condition; it's not a cure.

No matter which eating plan you and your doctor decide might be right for you, remember that you want a healthy, balanced diet to help your body work at its best. Your body needs protein, carbs, and fat to function properly. Your body, says Singh, needs a balanced diet, not one type of diet. It might be helpful for short-term weight loss but it might not be a long-term solution.

Bottom line: If a diet can help you manage your psoriatic arthritis with less medication, that's a good thing.

Psoriasis Arthritis Recipes

Here are a few simple, nutritious, delicious recipes to help start you on your new road to good health. Enjoy!

Trail Mix
Makes 8 to 10 servings

This snack or breakfast takes minutes to toss together and it's easy to take with you if you're in a rush. It's packed with nutrition and fibre to keep you going on your busiest days.

Ingredients

- 1 cup (250 mL) sliced almonds or chopped cashews
- 1 cup (250 mL) chopped walnuts
- 1 cup (250 mL) additive-free whole grain cereal of your choice
- ½ cup (125 mL) ground flax seeds
- ½ cup (125 mL) unsalted sunflower or pumpkin seeds
- 1 cup (250 mL) additive-free dried fruit
- 1 Tbsp (15 mL) cinnamon (optional)

Direction

1. Mix all ingredients together in a bowl
2. Store in an airtight container in the refrigerator until ready to use.

3. If you have diabetes and your daily routine makes it hard for you to eat regularly, try creating an emergency snack kit. Buy a fanny pack that you can attach to your waist or a small lunch bag that you can keep in your office or in your briefcase and fill it with diabetic-friendly snacks, such as an apple and peanut butter, trail mix, a small nut butter sandwich on 100% whole grain bread, or yogurt and chopped fruit.

Greens Smoothie
Serves 1 or 2

Who doesn't like a milkshake? This healthy version of this classic treat will satisfy your body as well as your soul.

Ingredients

- 1 cup whole milk, unsweetened almond or rice milk
- 1 cup fresh or frozen chopped fruit
- 2 tbsp additive-free peanut butter, almond butter or cashew butter

- 1 handful dark green leafy vegetables, such as spinach or kale
- Drizzle of honey (optional)

Direction

1. Put ingredients in a blender.
2. Blend until smooth.

Yogurt Sundae

This decadent indulgence makes a wonderful dessert that still has lots of nutritional value. Have some extra fun by letting your guests or family put together their own personalized sundaes.

Ingredients

- 1 cup (250 mL) full-fat plain yogurt
- 1 lightly sautéed chopped banana or 1 cup (250 mL) lightly sautéed chopped figs or mango
- 3 squares of dark chocolate, chopped
- A sprinkle of chopped nuts
- Honey or maple syrup to taste

Direction

1. Place the yogurt, fruit and chocolate in alternating layers in a bowl or sundae glass.
2. Top with chopped nuts and honey or maple syrup.

Almond Flour Cakes
Makes 12 mini-cakes

Satisfy your baked good cravings with these cakes, which are rich in both flavour and nutrition. The almond flour can help lower your cholesterol, while the cinnamon helps to stabilize your blood sugar but you and your guests will only be thinking about how good they taste!

Ingredients

- 2 cups (500 mL) finely ground almond flour
- Up to 1 Tbsp (15 mL) cinnamon
- ½ tsp (2 mL) baking soda
- Pinch salt
- 1 very ripe mashed banana
- 2 tsp (10 mL) pure vanilla extract

- 3 large eggs
- 1 cup (250 mL) chopped fresh or frozen fruit or berries (e.g., apple, blueberries, strawberries, banana)
- Chopped pecans (optional)

Direction

- Preheat the oven to 325°F (160°C) and line a muffin tin with paper baking cups.
- Mix the almond flour, cinnamon, baking soda, and salt in a bowl.
- Add the mashed banana, vanilla, and eggs to the flour mixture and whisk together until combined thoroughly and smooth.
- Stir in the berries or chopped fruit until they are distributed evenly throughout the batter.
- Scoop the batter into the prepared muffin tin and sprinkle the chopped pecans if desired. Bake until a knife comes out clean when inserted, about 18 to 20 minutes.
- Let cool.

Baked Rainbow Trout
Serves 3

Rich in anti-inflammatory omega-3 fats, this rainbow trout dish is the ultimate in healthy "fast food." It takes minutes to prepare and minutes to bake.

Ingredients

- ½ lb fillet rainbow trout
- 2 tsp (10 mL) olive oil
- 2 tsp (10 mL) dried herbs or 2 Tbsp (30 mL) chopped fresh herbs, such as chives, lemon balm, dill, thyme, tarragon, basil or parsley
- A sprinkle or two of salt and pepper
- Lemon wedges

Direction

1. Preheat the oven to 400°F (200°C).
2. Place the trout skin-side down in a glass baking dish and place the rest of the ingredients on top of the fish.

3. Rub the oil, herbs, salt and pepper evenly over both sides of the trout.
4. Bake the fish for 8 to 15 minutes, until the flesh is opaque and flakes easily when poked by a fork.
5. Serve with a large green salad, lightly sautéed spinach or grated beets, baked squash and some quinoa. Squeeze the juice from a wedge of lemon over the fish, if desired. Store leftovers in the refrigerator for up to 4 days and them to make a cold fish salad eaten on 100% whole-grain bread or a bed of dark leafy greens.

Baked Chicken
Serves 4

This savoury baked chicken features the anti-inflammatory spice turmeric, but can be made plainer if you're not a fan of its more exotic flavours. A sprinkle of salt and pepper and a drizzle of olive oil are all you need to make a quick and satisfying baked chicken meal.

Ingredients

- 1 Tbsp (15 mL) turmeric

- 1 Tbsp (15 mL) cumin
- 1 Tbsp (15 mL) paprika
- ½ tsp (2 mL) ground black pepper
- 1 tsp (5 mL) salt
- 2 lbs (1 kg) chicken legs
- 1 head cauliflower, chopped into florets
- 2 Tbsp (30 mL) olive or coconut oil

Direction

1. Preheat the oven to 350°F.
2. Mix the turmeric, cumin, paprika, pepper and salt in a bowl and stir until combined thoroughly.
3. Place the chicken and cauliflower in a large casserole dish and sprinkle them evenly with the spice mix.
4. Drizzle the olive or coconut oil over the chicken, cauliflower and spices.
5. Using your hands, rub the spices and oil into the chicken and cauliflower.
6. Bake for 45 to 60 minutes, until the chicken reaches an internal temperature of 180°F. Serve

hot and save leftovers for up to 4 days in the refrigerator for making sandwiches, salads and soups.

Gluten-Free Bean Salad
Serves 4

If you'd like to try a vegan meal, a classic rice and bean salad is a good place to start. Here is a basic recipe that you can try when you're feeling adventurous. Serve with a large green salad.

Ingredients

- 3 cups (750 mL) beans, drained and rinsed
- 2 Tbsp (30 mL) minced onions or scallions
- 1 garlic clove, pressed
- Salt and freshly ground pepper to taste
- ¼ cup (60 mL) fresh herbs, such as parsley, cilantro, basil, thyme, oregano or sage
- 2 Tbsp (30 mL) cold-pressed flax or olive oil
- Add 2 cups (500 mL) cooked brown rice or quinoa to make this into a meal (optional)

Direction

1. Put all the ingredients in a bowl and toss until thoroughly mixed.
2. Adjust seasoning to taste and store in the refrigerator in an airtight container until ready to serve.
3. Gluten is found in certain grains, such as wheat, rye, spelt, kamut and barley. But if you can't eat gluten, there are lots of gluten-free grains to choose from, such as corn, rice, quinoa, buckwheat, millet and amaranth. Oats are also naturally gluten-free, but tend to be processed on equipment that comes into contact with gluten-containing grains. If you want to eat oats, you must find a manufacturer that mills pure, uncontaminated oats.

Salad Dressing

1. Many store-bought salad dressings have unhealthy additives, such as MSG, stabilizers and sugar. As you can see from the recipe below, it's actually quite easy (and a lot cheaper) to make

your own salad dressing, so give it a try and experiment with different herbs until you find the flavours you like.

2. 1/3 cup (75 mL) cold-pressed flax oil, walnut oil or olive oil (see More Info box to find out more about oils and fats in your kitchen)
3. 2 Tbsp (30 mL) balsamic vinegar, lemon juice or apple cider vinegar
4. Chopped fresh herbs (optional)
5. Salt and pepper to taste
6. Put all the ingredients into a clean jar, close the lid and shake vigorously until the oil and vinegar have emulsified.
7. Pour over a dark leafy green salad, but not until you're ready to eat. Dressing the salad in advance will make it mushy and limp. Store in the fridge if you have leftovers and shake before using.

Apple and Onion Soup

6 servings

Ingredients

1 Tbsp canola oil

2 medium yellow onions, sliced

1 small leek, chopped

1/2 Tbsp fresh rosemary, chopped

1/2 Tbsp fresh thyme

3 organic apples, cut into small dices

6 cups fat-free, low-sodium vegetable broth

Directions

Heat the oil in a medium saucepan over medium heat. Add the onions and sauté until golden.

Pour in the broth and bring to the boil over medium-high heat. Add the apples, and reduce the heat to medium-low. Simmer for 10 minutes.

9. Zoodles with Mashed Avocado and Mediterranean Herbs

Serves 1

This Mediterranean-inspired recipe pairs zoodles with mashed avocado, garlic and Mediterranean herbs to create a creamy noodle-like dish that's full of flavor, antioxidants and essential fatty acids. Never heard of zoodles? Zoodles are basically just zucchini (courgette) cut into extra-thin, noodle-like strips. Naturally gluten-free, these imitation noodles make a great alternative to pasta for people who react adversely to grains and for those who follow a Paleo diet or another grain-free diet.

Note: This recipe uses yellow zucchini, which looks more like real noodles, but you can also use green zucchini to create this dish.

Ingredients

- 1 clove garlic
- Handful of fresh basil and oregano
- 1 avocado
- 1 yellow zucchini
- 1 Tbsp extra-virgin olive oil
- 1/4 cup water
- Salt, to taste

Directions

1. Peel and chop the garlic, and set it aside while you prepare the rest of the ingredients. Preparing the garlic before the other ingredients helps improve its health benefits as allicin, the key active ingredient in garlic, takes some time to form after peeling and chopping.

2. Rinse and chop the herbs and set them aside.
3. Peel the avocado and remove the pit. Place the peeled and pitted avocado in a small bowl and mash thoroughly with a fork. Set aside.
4. Wash the zucchini under cold running water, and cut it into long, thin noodle-shaped slices (zoodles) using a sturdy vegetable spiralizer, julienne slicer or electric zoodle maker. Set aside.
5. Heat the olive oil in a skillet and saute the chopped garlic over medium heat for 1 minute. Add the zoodles and continue to saute for another minute or two, stirring frequently.
6. Add the water and continue cooking for 4 more minutes, stirring occasionally.
7. Remove the skillet from the heat, and let it cool slightly. Stir in the avocado, chopped herbs and salt, and serve immediately.

Wholesome Winter Pea and Watercress Soup

6 servings

Ingredients

- 1 large onion
- 1 garlic clove
- 6 cups vegetable or chicken stock
- 1 zucchini
- 30 oz frozen peas
- 3 oz watercress
- Salt and pepper, to taste

Directions

1. Peel and crush the garlic and set aside. Leaving crushed or minced garlic for at least 5-10 minutes after crushing helps maximize its health-protective effects.
2. While health-promoting compounds are forming in crushed garlic, wash and trim the zucchini, and cut it into chunks.

3. Peel and chop the onion, and sweat it, together with the minced garlic, in 2-3 tablespoons of chicken or vegetable stock in a stock pot.
4. Add the zucchini chunks and pour in the rest of the stock. Bring to a boil and simmer for until the zucchini chunks are just cooked, about 10 minutes.
5. Add the frozen peas and simmer for 3 minutes. Add the watercress and simmer for another minute.
6. Remove from the heat and let cool for a few minutes. Process with a hand-held blender until smooth. Season with salt.

Broccoli and Barley Soup
6 servings

Ingredients

- 1/4 cup yellow onion, chopped
- 1 small carrot, peeled and diced
- 1 rib organic celery, finely chopped
- 1 tbsp extra virgin olive oil

- 4 cups small, organic broccoli florets
- 1/2 cup pearled barley, cooked
- 5 cups vegetable broth
- 1 can (14 1/2 oz) stewed tomatoes
- 4 cloves garlic, minced
- 1/4 tsp dried marjoram
- 1 tsp thyme
- Salt and pepper, to taste

Directions

1. In a stock pot, cook onion in olive oil over medium heat for 4-5 minutes until soft.
2. Add vegetable broth and bring to a boil. Reduce to a simmer and add celery and carrots along with broccoli florets. Cover and let simmer until carrots and broccoli florets are tender.
3. Add cooked barley, canned tomatoes, garlic, marjoram, and thyme. Let simmer another minute or two.
4. Season with salt and pepper. Serve warm.

Chicken Soup with Rice and Broccoli
6 servings

Ingredients

- 4 cups fat-free, low-sodium chicken broth
- 1 small onion, chopped
- 1 1/2 cups broccoli florets
- 2 small ribs organic celery, diced
- 2 small carrots, sliced
- 1/2 cup short grain brown rice, washed
- 2 cups cooked, skinless chicken, diced

Directions

1. Soak rice in cold water from 15 minutes to one hour. This will reduce cooking time.
2. Bring broth to a boil in a large saucepan. Add presoaked rice and vegetables. Reduce heat to low, cover and simmer, stirring occasionally, until rice is tender.
3. Add cooked chicken and simmer for 3-4 minutes.

Chicken and Apple Salad

Serves 4

Ingredients

- 3 cups cooked chicken, diced
- 1 cup grapes, halved
- 1/2 cup celery, diced
- 3 tbsp red onion, finely chopped
- 1/2 cup organic apples, diced
- 6 tbsp extra light mayonnaise
- 2 tsp lemon juice
- Salt and pepper, to taste
- Lettuce leaves

Directions

1. Combine first five ingredients in a large bowl.
2. In a small bowl, combine mayonnaise, lemon juice, and salt and pepper. Stir into chicken mix.
3. Arrange lettuce leaves on serving plates and top with chicken salad.

Broccoli Salad with Apples and Cranberries

6 servings

This low-GI broccoli salad featuring apples and cranberries is low in calories and low in fat, but loaded with a wide range of nutrients.

Ingredients

- 4 cups fresh broccoli florets
- 1/2 cup dried cranberries
- 1/2 cup sunflower seeds
- 3 organic apples
- 1/4 cup red onion, chopped
- 1 cup plain, low-fat yoghurt with probiotic bacteria
- 2 Tbsp Dijon style mustard
- 1/4 cup honey

Directions

1. Combine broccoli florets, dried cranberries, sunflower seeds, chopped apples, and chopped

onion in a large serving bowl. Blend yoghurt, mustard, and honey in a small bowl.
2. Add dressing to the salad and toss. Chill before serving.

Romaine and Smoked Salmon Salad
Serves 2

Ingredients

- 1 small head organic romaine lettuce
- 5 ounces smoked salmon, thinly sliced
- 2 tomatoes, diced
- 4 radishes, thinly sliced
- 1 organic carrot, diagonally sliced
- 1/2 cucumber, peeled and diced
- Juice of half a lemon
- 1 tsp fresh ginger root, peeled and minced
- 1 tbsp canola oil

Directions

1. Arrange romaine lettuce on two plates. Top with salmon, tomatoes, radishes, carrots, and cucumber.
2. Shake lemon juice, canola oil, and minced ginger in tightly covered jar. Pour over salad.

Beet and Carrot Salad with Ginger
Serves 1

Ingredients

- 1/2 cup raw beets, peeled and grated
- 1/2 cup organic carrots, grated
- 2 tbsp apple juice
- 1 tbsp extra-virgin olive oil
- 1/2 tsp fresh ginger, minced
- 1/8 tsp sea salt

Directions

1. Combine grated beets and carrots in a small bowl.
2. Mix apple juice, olive oil, ginger, and salt in a separate bowl and drizzle over salad mixture. Toss gently. Enjoy

Beet and Carrot Soup
Serves 4

Ingredients

- 3 medium beets, peeled and diced
- 1 tbsp olive oil
- 1 cup onion, chopped
- 1 pound carrots, diced
- 1 tbsp fresh ginger, minced
- 1 garlic clove, minced
- 6 cups vegetable stock

Directions

1. Heat oil in a large saucepan over medium heat. Sauté onion until golden brown. Add ginger and garlic and cook for 2 minutes, stirring frequently.
2. Add beets, carrots, and stock. Reduce heat to low and simmer covered until beets and carrots are tender, about 25 minutes.
3. In a food processor, purée soup in batches. Taste soup and adjust seasonings.
4. Serve hot or cold, garnished with cilantro leaves.

Omega-3 Omelet with Red Onions and Capers

3 servings

Ingredients

- 4 large omega-3 enriched eggs
- 1 red onion, chopped
- 3 tsp capers
- 2 tbsp extra virgin olive oil
- 1 1/2 tbsp water
- 1/4 tsp salt

Directions

1. Grease a non-stick frying pan with a paper towel dipped in extra-virgin olive oil. Add onion fry until almost golden.
2. Beat eggs, water, and salt together in a small bowl. Add capers to mixture and pour over onions.
3. Cook until egg is just set. Turn omelet over once.
4. Transfer omelet onto a plate. Garnish as desired.

Barley Soup with Carrots and Parsley
2 servings

Ingredients

- 2/3 cup water
- 1/3 cup pearled barley
- 2 tbsp extra virgin olive oil
- 1/2 cup yellow onion, chopped
- 1 cup carrots
- 2 cups vegetable stock
- 1 2/3 cup plain yogurt containing probiotic bacteria
- 2/3 cup fresh parsley, minced
- Salt and pepper, to taste
- 1/2 tsp black pepper, freshly ground

Directions

1. Bring water to a boil in a soup pot. Add barley and let simmer covered for about 25-30 minutes over low heat. Once water has evaporated, remove from heat and set aside

2. In a stock pot, cook onion in olive oil over medium heat for 4-5 minutes until soft. Add stock and carrots and bring to boil. Reduce to a simmer, cover, and cook for 20 minutes.
3. Add cooked barley and let simmer another minute or two. Remove from heat.
4. Stir in yoghurt and seasonings. Serve immediately.

Conclusion

Psoriasis is a very troublesome disease with a high economic impact. The disease often persists for life, and the patient has an increased risk of cardiovascular diseases and their complications. One out of five patients develops psoriatic arthritis. The clinical picture of psoriasis is highly variable with regard to lesional characteristics and the severity of disease. To improve the management of psoriasis the guidelines must be followed and all appropriate topical and systemic treatment options must be tried, with clearly defined treatment goals. The spectrum of established systemic treatments for psoriasis has been extended by the biologics. These can be used to achieve a good skin status and a clear-cut improvement in quality of life even in patients who do not or no longer respond adequately to conventional therapies.